# BLOOD PREASURE LOG BOOK

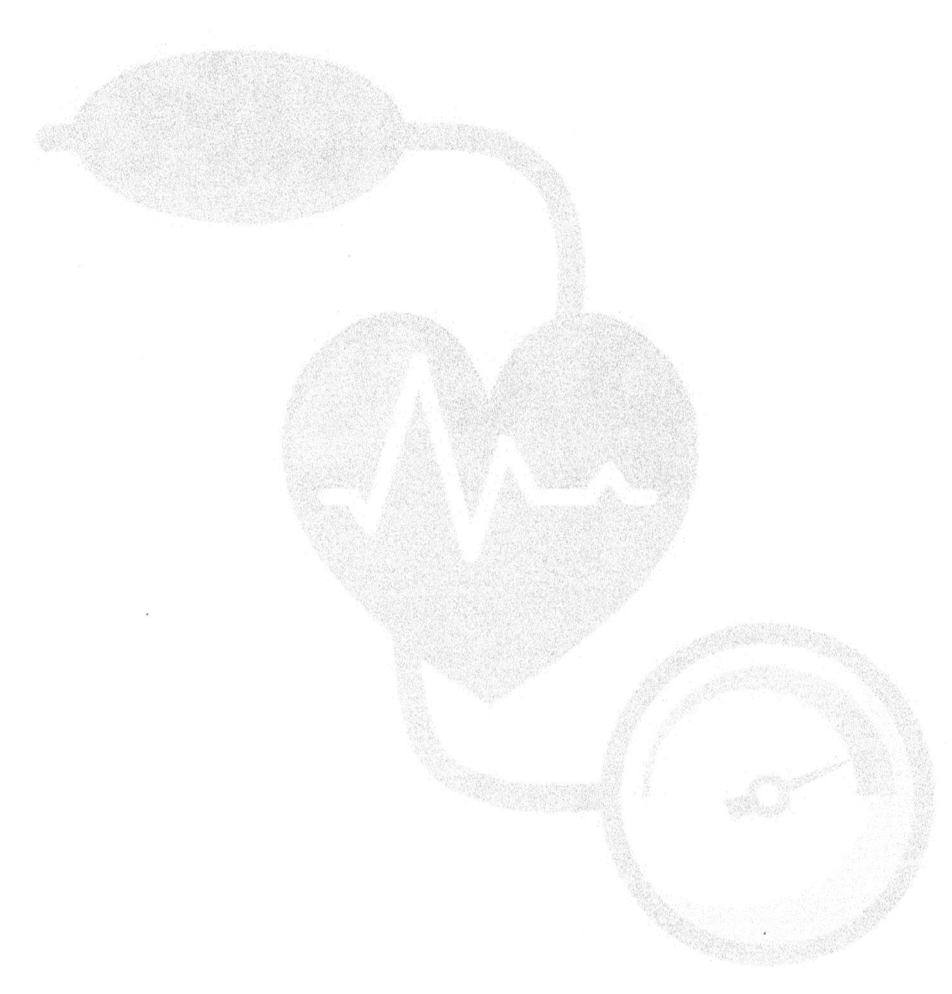

# Reference Values

| Blood Pressure | Systolic mm Hg (upper number) | Diastolic mm Hg (upper number) |
|---|---|---|
| Normal | Less than 120 | Less than 80 |
| Elevated | 120 - 129 | Less than 80 |
| High blood pressure (hypertension stage I) | 130 - 139 | 80 - 89 |
| High blood pressure (hypertension stage II) | 140 or higher | 90 or higher |
| Hypertensive crisis (consult doctor immediately) | Higher than 180 | Higher than 120 |

Date .............................................................................................................................

Sleep quality and duration ...............................................................................................

Stress levels        1     2     3     4     5     6     7     8     9     10

| Time | Systolic | Diastolic | Heart Rate |
|---|---|---|---|
|  |  |  |  |
|  |  |  |  |
|  |  |  |  |
|  |  |  |  |
|  |  |  |  |

Exercise and daily activities                    Water Intake

| Breakfast | Lunch |
|---|---|
|  |  |

| Dinner | Snacks |
|---|---|
|  |  |

| Supplements | Medication |
|---|---|
|  |  |

Date  ....................................................................................................................

Sleep quality and duration  ...............................................................................

Stress levels      1    2    3    4    5    6    7    8    9    10

| Time | Systolic | Diastolic | Heart Rate |
|------|----------|-----------|------------|
|      |          |           |            |
|      |          |           |            |
|      |          |           |            |
|      |          |           |            |
|      |          |           |            |

Exercise and daily activities        Water Intake

| Breakfast | Lunch |
|-----------|-------|
|           |       |

| Dinner | Snacks |
|--------|--------|
|        |        |

| Supplements | Medication |
|-------------|------------|
|             |            |

Date ..............................................................................................

Sleep quality and duration ...........................................................

Stress levels     1   2   3   4   5   6   7   8   9   10

| Time | Systolic | Diastolic | Heart Rate |
|---|---|---|---|
|  |  |  |  |
|  |  |  |  |
|  |  |  |  |
|  |  |  |  |
|  |  |  |  |

## Exercise and daily activities

Water Intake ▢▢▢▢▢▢▢

..............................................................
..............................................................
..............................................................
..............................................................
..............................................................
..............................................................
..............................................................
..............................................................
..............................................................
..............................................................
..............................................................
..............................................................
..............................................................
..............................................................
..............................................................

| Breakfast | Lunch |
|---|---|
|  |  |

| Dinner | Snacks |
|---|---|
|  |  |

| Supplements | Medication |
|---|---|
|  |  |

Date ...............................................................................................................

Sleep quality and duration ............................................................................

Stress levels      1    2    3    4    5    6    7    8    9    10

| Time | Systolic | Diastolic | Heart Rate |
|------|----------|-----------|------------|
|      |          |           |            |
|      |          |           |            |
|      |          |           |            |
|      |          |           |            |
|      |          |           |            |

**Exercise and daily activities**        **Water Intake**

| Breakfast | Lunch |
|-----------|-------|
|           |       |

| Dinner | Snacks |
|--------|--------|
|        |        |

| Supplements | Medication |
|-------------|------------|
|             |            |

Date ......................................................................................................

Sleep quality and duration ............................................................................

Stress levels          1     2     3     4     5     6     7     8     9     10

| Time | Systolic | Diastolic | Heart Rate |
|------|----------|-----------|------------|
|      |          |           |            |
|      |          |           |            |
|      |          |           |            |
|      |          |           |            |
|      |          |           |            |

Exercise and daily activities          Water Intake

| Breakfast | Lunch |
|-----------|-------|
|           |       |

| Dinner | Snacks |
|--------|--------|
|        |        |

| Supplements | Medication |
|-------------|------------|
|             |            |

Date .................................................................................................

Sleep quality and duration ................................................................

Stress levels     1    2    3    4    5    6    7    8    9    10

| Time | Systolic | Diastolic | Heart Rate |
|------|----------|-----------|------------|
|      |          |           |            |
|      |          |           |            |
|      |          |           |            |
|      |          |           |            |
|      |          |           |            |

Exercise and daily activities        Water Intake

| Breakfast | Lunch |
|-----------|-------|
|           |       |

| Dinner | Snacks |
|--------|--------|
|        |        |

| Supplements | Medication |
|-------------|------------|
|             |            |

Date ....................................................................................................................

Sleep quality and duration ...............................................................................

Stress levels      1    2    3    4    5    6    7    8    9    10

| Time | Systolic | Diastolic | Heart Rate |
|------|----------|-----------|------------|
|      |          |           |            |
|      |          |           |            |
|      |          |           |            |
|      |          |           |            |
|      |          |           |            |

Exercise and daily activities      Water Intake

| Breakfast | Lunch |
|-----------|-------|
|           |       |

| Dinner | Snacks |
|--------|--------|
|        |        |

| Supplements | Medication |
|-------------|------------|
|             |            |

Date ...............................................................................................

Sleep quality and duration ...............................................................

Stress levels      1    2    3    4    5    6    7    8    9    10

| Time | Systolic | Diastolic | Heart Rate |
|---|---|---|---|
|  |  |  |  |
|  |  |  |  |
|  |  |  |  |
|  |  |  |  |
|  |  |  |  |

Exercise and daily activities          Water Intake

| Breakfast | Lunch |
|---|---|
|  |  |

| Dinner | Snacks |
|---|---|
|  |  |

| Supplements | Medication |
|---|---|
|  |  |

Date ............................................................................................................

Sleep quality and duration ...................................................................................

Stress levels     1    2    3    4    5    6    7    8    9    10

| Time | Systolic | Diastolic | Heart Rate |
|---|---|---|---|
|  |  |  |  |
|  |  |  |  |
|  |  |  |  |
|  |  |  |  |
|  |  |  |  |

Exercise and daily activities      Water Intake

...........................................................

...........................................................

...........................................................

...........................................................

...........................................................

...........................................................

...........................................................

...........................................................

...........................................................

...........................................................

...........................................................

...........................................................

...........................................................

...........................................................

| Breakfast | Lunch |
|---|---|
|  |  |

| Dinner | Snacks |
|---|---|
|  |  |

| Supplements | Medication |
|---|---|
|  |  |

Date  .................................................................................................

Sleep quality and duration  ...........................................................

Stress levels      1    2    3    4    5    6    7    8    9    10

| Time | Systolic | Diastolic | Heart Rate |
|---|---|---|---|
|  |  |  |  |
|  |  |  |  |
|  |  |  |  |
|  |  |  |  |

**Exercise and daily activities**

**Water Intake**

| Breakfast | Lunch |
|---|---|
|  |  |

| Dinner | Snacks |
|---|---|
|  |  |

| Supplements | Medication |
|---|---|
|  |  |

Date  ...........................................................................................................................

Sleep quality and duration  ...........................................................................................

Stress levels     1     2     3     4     5     6     7     8     9     10

| Time | Systolic | Diastolic | Heart Rate |
| --- | --- | --- | --- |
|  |  |  |  |
|  |  |  |  |
|  |  |  |  |
|  |  |  |  |
|  |  |  |  |

Exercise and daily activities

Water Intake ▯▯▯▯▯▯▯

| Breakfast | Lunch |
| --- | --- |
|  |  |

| Dinner | Snacks |
| --- | --- |
|  |  |

| Supplements | Medication |
| --- | --- |
|  |  |

Date .................................................................................................

Sleep quality and duration .........................................................

Stress levels     1   2   3   4   5   6   7   8   9   10

| Time | Systolic | Diastolic | Heart Rate |
|------|----------|-----------|------------|
|      |          |           |            |
|      |          |           |            |
|      |          |           |            |
|      |          |           |            |
|      |          |           |            |

Exercise and daily activities        Water Intake

| Breakfast | Lunch |
|-----------|-------|
|           |       |
| Dinner | Snacks |
|        |        |
| Supplements | Medication |
|             |            |

Date .......................................................................................................

Sleep quality and duration .................................................................

Stress levels      1    2    3    4    5    6    7    8    9    10

| Time | Systolic | Diastolic | Heart Rate |
|------|----------|-----------|------------|
|      |          |           |            |
|      |          |           |            |
|      |          |           |            |
|      |          |           |            |
|      |          |           |            |

**Exercise and daily activities**        Water Intake ☐☐☐☐☐☐☐

....................................................................
....................................................................
....................................................................
....................................................................
....................................................................
....................................................................
....................................................................
....................................................................
....................................................................
....................................................................
....................................................................
....................................................................
....................................................................
....................................................................

| Breakfast | Lunch |
|-----------|-------|
|           |       |

| Dinner | Snacks |
|--------|--------|
|        |        |

| Supplements | Medication |
|-------------|------------|
|             |            |

Date  ......................................................................................

Sleep quality and duration  ................................................................

Stress levels       1    2    3    4    5    6    7    8    9    10

| Time | Systolic | Diastolic | Heart Rate |
|---|---|---|---|
|  |  |  |  |
|  |  |  |  |
|  |  |  |  |
|  |  |  |  |
|  |  |  |  |

Exercise and daily activities      Water Intake

| Breakfast | Lunch |
|---|---|
|  |  |
| Dinner | Snacks |
|  |  |
| Supplements | Medication |
|  |  |

Date .................................................................................................................

Sleep quality and duration ...........................................................................

Stress levels     1   2   3   4   5   6   7   8   9   10

| Time | Systolic | Diastolic | Heart Rate |
|------|----------|-----------|------------|
|      |          |           |            |
|      |          |           |            |
|      |          |           |            |
|      |          |           |            |
|      |          |           |            |

Exercise and daily activities     Water Intake

.....................................................................
.....................................................................
.....................................................................
.....................................................................
.....................................................................
.....................................................................
.....................................................................
.....................................................................
.....................................................................
.....................................................................
.....................................................................
.....................................................................
.....................................................................
.....................................................................
.....................................................................

| Breakfast | Lunch |
|-----------|-------|
|           |       |

| Dinner | Snacks |
|--------|--------|
|        |        |

| Supplements | Medication |
|-------------|------------|
|             |            |

Date ..........................................................................................

Sleep quality and duration ...................................................................

Stress levels      1   2   3   4   5   6   7   8   9   10

| Time | Systolic | Diastolic | Heart Rate |
|------|----------|-----------|------------|
|      |          |           |            |
|      |          |           |            |
|      |          |           |            |
|      |          |           |            |
|      |          |           |            |

Exercise and daily activities      Water Intake

....................................................

....................................................

....................................................

....................................................

....................................................

....................................................

....................................................

....................................................

....................................................

....................................................

....................................................

....................................................

....................................................

....................................................

| Breakfast | Lunch |
|-----------|-------|
|           |       |

| Dinner | Snacks |
|--------|--------|
|        |        |

| Supplements | Medication |
|-------------|------------|
|             |            |

Date .................................................................................................

Sleep quality and duration ...........................................................

Stress levels     1   2   3   4   5   6   7   8   9   10

| Time | Systolic | Diastolic | Heart Rate |
|------|----------|-----------|------------|
|      |          |           |            |
|      |          |           |            |
|      |          |           |            |
|      |          |           |            |
|      |          |           |            |

Exercise and daily activities     Water Intake

| Breakfast | Lunch |
|-----------|-------|
|           |       |

| Dinner | Snacks |
|--------|--------|
|        |        |

| Supplements | Medication |
|-------------|------------|
|             |            |

Date ............................................................................................................

Sleep quality and duration ...................................................................

Stress levels     1    2    3    4    5    6    7    8    9    10

| Time | Systolic | Diastolic | Heart Rate |
|------|----------|-----------|------------|
|      |          |           |            |
|      |          |           |            |
|      |          |           |            |
|      |          |           |            |
|      |          |           |            |

Exercise and daily activities      Water Intake

| Breakfast | Lunch |
|-----------|-------|
|           |       |

| Dinner | Snacks |
|--------|--------|
|        |        |

| Supplements | Medication |
|-------------|------------|
|             |            |

Date ...........................................................................................................................

Sleep quality and duration ...................................................................................

Stress levels        1    2    3    4    5    6    7    8    9    10

| Time | Systolic | Diastolic | Heart Rate |
|---|---|---|---|
|  |  |  |  |
|  |  |  |  |
|  |  |  |  |
|  |  |  |  |
|  |  |  |  |

Exercise and daily activities      Water Intake

...........................................................................

...........................................................................

...........................................................................

...........................................................................

...........................................................................

...........................................................................

...........................................................................

...........................................................................

...........................................................................

...........................................................................

...........................................................................

...........................................................................

...........................................................................

...........................................................................

...........................................................................

| Breakfast | Lunch |
|---|---|
|  |  |

| Dinner | Snacks |
|---|---|
|  |  |

| Supplements | Medication |
|---|---|
|  |  |

Date ..................................................................................

Sleep quality and duration  ...............................................

Stress levels     1   2   3   4   5   6   7   8   9   10

| Time | Systolic | Diastolic | Heart Rate |
|---|---|---|---|
|  |  |  |  |
|  |  |  |  |
|  |  |  |  |
|  |  |  |  |
|  |  |  |  |

**Exercise and daily activities**      Water Intake

| Breakfast | Lunch |
|---|---|
|  |  |
| Dinner | Snacks |
|  |  |
| Supplements | Medication |
|  |  |

Date  .........................................................................................................

Sleep quality and duration  ...............................................................

Stress levels        1     2     3     4     5     6     7     8     9     10

| Time | Systolic | Diastolic | Heart Rate |
|------|----------|-----------|------------|
|      |          |           |            |
|      |          |           |            |
|      |          |           |            |
|      |          |           |            |
|      |          |           |            |

Exercise and daily activities            Water Intake

| Breakfast | Lunch |
|-----------|-------|
|           |       |

| Dinner | Snacks |
|--------|--------|
|        |        |

| Supplements | Medication |
|-------------|------------|
|             |            |

Date .................................................................................

Sleep quality and duration .............................................................

Stress levels          1     2     3     4     5     6     7     8     9     10

| Time | Systolic | Diastolic | Heart Rate |
|------|----------|-----------|------------|
|      |          |           |            |
|      |          |           |            |
|      |          |           |            |
|      |          |           |            |
|      |          |           |            |

Exercise and daily activities          Water Intake

..............................................

..............................................

..............................................

..............................................

..............................................

..............................................

..............................................

..............................................

..............................................

..............................................

..............................................

..............................................

..............................................

| Breakfast | Lunch |
|-----------|-------|
|           |       |

| Dinner | Snacks |
|--------|--------|
|        |        |

| Supplements | Medication |
|-------------|------------|
|             |            |

Date .............................................................................................................

Sleep quality and duration ...........................................................................

Stress levels     1    2    3    4    5    6    7    8    9    10

| Time | Systolic | Diastolic | Heart Rate |
|---|---|---|---|
|  |  |  |  |
|  |  |  |  |
|  |  |  |  |
|  |  |  |  |
|  |  |  |  |

**Exercise and daily activities**     Water Intake

..............................................................

..............................................................

..............................................................

..............................................................

..............................................................

..............................................................

..............................................................

..............................................................

..............................................................

..............................................................

..............................................................

..............................................................

..............................................................

..............................................................

| Breakfast | Lunch |
|---|---|
|  |  |

| Dinner | Snacks |
|---|---|
|  |  |

| Supplements | Medication |
|---|---|
|  |  |

Date .................................................................................................

Sleep quality and duration .................................................................

Stress levels      1    2    3    4    5    6    7    8    9    10

| Time | Systolic | Diastolic | Heart Rate |
|---|---|---|---|
|  |  |  |  |
|  |  |  |  |
|  |  |  |  |
|  |  |  |  |
|  |  |  |  |

Exercise and daily activities      Water Intake

| Breakfast | Lunch |
|---|---|
|  |  |
| Dinner | Snacks |
|  |  |
| Supplements | Medication |
|  |  |

Date .......................................................................................................

Sleep quality and duration ...................................................................

Stress levels     1    2    3    4    5    6    7    8    9    10

| Time | Systolic | Diastolic | Heart Rate |
|------|----------|-----------|------------|
|      |          |           |            |
|      |          |           |            |
|      |          |           |            |
|      |          |           |            |
|      |          |           |            |

Exercise and daily activities      Water Intake

| Breakfast | Lunch |
|-----------|-------|
|           |       |

| Dinner | Snacks |
|--------|--------|
|        |        |

| Supplements | Medication |
|-------------|------------|
|             |            |

Date .................................................................................................................

Sleep quality and duration ......................................................................

Stress levels      1   2   3   4   5   6   7   8   9   10

| Time | Systolic | Diastolic | Heart Rate |
|------|----------|-----------|------------|
|      |          |           |            |
|      |          |           |            |
|      |          |           |            |
|      |          |           |            |
|      |          |           |            |

Exercise and daily activities      Water Intake

..............................................................

..............................................................

..............................................................

..............................................................

..............................................................

..............................................................

..............................................................

..............................................................

..............................................................

..............................................................

..............................................................

..............................................................

..............................................................

| Breakfast | Lunch |
|-----------|-------|
|           |       |

| Dinner | Snacks |
|--------|--------|
|        |        |

| Supplements | Medication |
|-------------|------------|
|             |            |

Date ...............................................................................................................

Sleep quality and duration ...................................................................................

Stress levels     1    2    3    4    5    6    7    8    9    10

| Time | Systolic | Diastolic | Heart Rate |
|---|---|---|---|
|  |  |  |  |
|  |  |  |  |
|  |  |  |  |
|  |  |  |  |
|  |  |  |  |

Exercise and daily activities      Water Intake

| Breakfast | Lunch |
|---|---|
|  |  |
| Dinner | Snacks |
|  |  |
| Supplements | Medication |
|  |  |

Date ................................................................................................................

Sleep quality and duration ....................................................................................

Stress levels      1    2    3    4    5    6    7    8    9    10

| Time | Systolic | Diastolic | Heart Rate |
|------|----------|-----------|------------|
|      |          |           |            |
|      |          |           |            |
|      |          |           |            |
|      |          |           |            |
|      |          |           |            |

Exercise and daily activities      Water Intake

| Breakfast | Lunch |
|-----------|-------|
|           |       |
| Dinner | Snacks |
|        |        |
| Supplements | Medication |
|             |            |

Date .................................................................................................................................

Sleep quality and duration .................................................................................................

Stress levels      1    2    3    4    5    6    7    8    9    10

| Time | Systolic | Diastolic | Heart Rate |
|------|----------|-----------|------------|
|      |          |           |            |
|      |          |           |            |
|      |          |           |            |
|      |          |           |            |
|      |          |           |            |

Exercise and daily activities        Water Intake   ☐ ☐ ☐ ☐ ☐ ☐ ☐

..............................................................

..............................................................

..............................................................

..............................................................

..............................................................

..............................................................

..............................................................

..............................................................

..............................................................

..............................................................

..............................................................

..............................................................

..............................................................

..............................................................

| Breakfast | Lunch |
|-----------|-------|
|           |       |

| Dinner | Snacks |
|--------|--------|
|        |        |

| Supplements | Medication |
|-------------|------------|
|             |            |

Date ...........................................................................................................

Sleep quality and duration .......................................................................

Stress levels      1    2    3    4    5    6    7    8    9    10

| Time | Systolic | Diastolic | Heart Rate |
|------|----------|-----------|------------|
|      |          |           |            |
|      |          |           |            |
|      |          |           |            |
|      |          |           |            |
|      |          |           |            |

Exercise and daily activities      Water Intake

| Breakfast | Lunch |
|-----------|-------|
|           |       |

| Dinner | Snacks |
|--------|--------|
|        |        |

| Supplements | Medication |
|-------------|------------|
|             |            |

Date .............................................................................................................

Sleep quality and duration ...................................................................

Stress levels      1    2    3    4    5    6    7    8    9    10

| Time | Systolic | Diastolic | Heart Rate |
|---|---|---|---|
|  |  |  |  |
|  |  |  |  |
|  |  |  |  |
|  |  |  |  |
|  |  |  |  |

Exercise and daily activities      Water Intake

..............................................................

..............................................................

..............................................................

..............................................................

..............................................................

..............................................................

..............................................................

..............................................................

..............................................................

..............................................................

..............................................................

..............................................................

..............................................................

..............................................................

| Breakfast | Lunch |
|---|---|
|  |  |

| Dinner | Snacks |
|---|---|
|  |  |

| Supplements | Medication |
|---|---|
|  |  |

Date .......................................................................................

Sleep quality and duration ..........................................................

Stress levels     1    2    3    4    5    6    7    8    9    10

| Time | Systolic | Diastolic | Heart Rate |
|------|----------|-----------|------------|
|      |          |           |            |
|      |          |           |            |
|      |          |           |            |
|      |          |           |            |
|      |          |           |            |

Exercise and daily activities     Water Intake

| Breakfast | Lunch |
|-----------|-------|
|           |       |

| Dinner | Snacks |
|--------|--------|
|        |        |

| Supplements | Medication |
|-------------|------------|
|             |            |

Date .............................................................................................................................

Sleep quality and duration ..................................................................................

Stress levels        1    2    3    4    5    6    7    8    9    10

| Time | Systolic | Diastolic | Heart Rate |
|------|----------|-----------|------------|
|      |          |           |            |
|      |          |           |            |
|      |          |           |            |
|      |          |           |            |
|      |          |           |            |

Exercise and daily activities          Water Intake

| Breakfast | Lunch |
|-----------|-------|
|           |       |

| Dinner | Snacks |
|--------|--------|
|        |        |

| Supplements | Medication |
|-------------|------------|
|             |            |

Date ............................................................................

Sleep quality and duration ....................................................

Stress levels     1   2   3   4   5   6   7   8   9   10

| Time | Systolic | Diastolic | Heart Rate |
|------|----------|-----------|------------|
|      |          |           |            |
|      |          |           |            |
|      |          |           |            |
|      |          |           |            |
|      |          |           |            |

Exercise and daily activities      Water Intake

...............................................

...............................................

...............................................

...............................................

...............................................

...............................................

...............................................

...............................................

...............................................

...............................................

...............................................

...............................................

...............................................

...............................................

| Breakfast | Lunch |
|-----------|-------|
|           |       |

| Dinner | Snacks |
|--------|--------|
|        |        |

| Supplements | Medication |
|-------------|------------|
|             |            |

Date .........................................................................................................................

Sleep quality and duration .......................................................................................

Stress levels       1    2    3    4    5    6    7    8    9    10

| Time | Systolic | Diastolic | Heart Rate |
|------|----------|-----------|------------|
|      |          |           |            |
|      |          |           |            |
|      |          |           |            |
|      |          |           |            |
|      |          |           |            |

**Exercise and daily activities**

.............................................................
.............................................................
.............................................................
.............................................................
.............................................................
.............................................................
.............................................................
.............................................................
.............................................................
.............................................................
.............................................................
.............................................................
.............................................................
.............................................................
.............................................................

Water Intake ☐ ☐ ☐ ☐ ☐ ☐ ☐

| Breakfast | Lunch |
|-----------|-------|
|           |       |

| Dinner | Snacks |
|--------|--------|
|        |        |

| Supplements | Medication |
|-------------|------------|
|             |            |

Date .............................................................................................

Sleep quality and duration .............................................................

Stress levels     1    2    3    4    5    6    7    8    9    10

| Time | Systolic | Diastolic | Heart Rate |
|------|----------|-----------|------------|
|      |          |           |            |
|      |          |           |            |
|      |          |           |            |
|      |          |           |            |
|      |          |           |            |

Exercise and daily activities      Water Intake ☐ ☐ ☐ ☐ ☐ ☐ ☐

| Breakfast | Lunch |
|-----------|-------|
|           |       |

| Dinner | Snacks |
|--------|--------|
|        |        |

| Supplements | Medication |
|-------------|------------|
|             |            |

Date ................................................................................................................

Sleep quality and duration ...................................................................................

Stress levels      1    2    3    4    5    6    7    8    9    10

| Time | Systolic | Diastolic | Heart Rate |
|------|----------|-----------|------------|
|      |          |           |            |
|      |          |           |            |
|      |          |           |            |
|      |          |           |            |
|      |          |           |            |

**Exercise and daily activities**      **Water Intake** ☐ ☐ ☐ ☐ ☐ ☐ ☐

| Breakfast | Lunch |
|-----------|-------|
|           |       |

| Dinner | Snacks |
|--------|--------|
|        |        |

| Supplements | Medication |
|-------------|------------|
|             |            |

Date .........................................................................................................

Sleep quality and duration .....................................................................

Stress levels     1    2    3    4    5    6    7    8    9    10

| Time | Systolic | Diastolic | Heart Rate |
|------|----------|-----------|------------|
|      |          |           |            |
|      |          |           |            |
|      |          |           |            |
|      |          |           |            |
|      |          |           |            |

Exercise and daily activities      Water Intake

......................................................

......................................................

......................................................

......................................................

......................................................

......................................................

......................................................

......................................................

......................................................

......................................................

......................................................

......................................................

......................................................

| Breakfast | Lunch |
|-----------|-------|
|           |       |

| Dinner | Snacks |
|--------|--------|
|        |        |

| Supplements | Medication |
|-------------|------------|
|             |            |

Date ...........................................................................................................

Sleep quality and duration ..................................................................

Stress levels        1    2    3    4    5    6    7    8    9    10

| Time | Systolic | Diastolic | Heart Rate |
|------|----------|-----------|------------|
|      |          |           |            |
|      |          |           |            |
|      |          |           |            |
|      |          |           |            |
|      |          |           |            |

Exercise and daily activities          Water Intake

..............................................

..............................................

..............................................

..............................................

..............................................

..............................................

..............................................

..............................................

..............................................

..............................................

..............................................

..............................................

..............................................

..............................................

..............................................

| Breakfast | Lunch |
|-----------|-------|
|           |       |

| Dinner | Snacks |
|--------|--------|
|        |        |

| Supplements | Medication |
|-------------|------------|
|             |            |

Date ....................................................................................................

Sleep quality and duration ...................................................................

Stress levels     1   2   3   4   5   6   7   8   9   10

| Time | Systolic | Diastolic | Heart Rate |
| --- | --- | --- | --- |
|  |  |  |  |
|  |  |  |  |
|  |  |  |  |
|  |  |  |  |
|  |  |  |  |

Exercise and daily activities      Water Intake

| Breakfast | Lunch |
| --- | --- |
|  |  |
| Dinner | Snacks |
|  |  |
| Supplements | Medication |
|  |  |

Date ...........................................................................................................

Sleep quality and duration ...................................................................

Stress levels      1    2    3    4    5    6    7    8    9    10

| Time | Systolic | Diastolic | Heart Rate |
|------|----------|-----------|------------|
|      |          |           |            |
|      |          |           |            |
|      |          |           |            |
|      |          |           |            |
|      |          |           |            |

Exercise and daily activities      Water Intake

..............................................................

..............................................................

..............................................................

..............................................................

..............................................................

..............................................................

..............................................................

..............................................................

..............................................................

..............................................................

..............................................................

..............................................................

..............................................................

..............................................................

| Breakfast | Lunch |
|-----------|-------|
|           |       |

| Dinner | Snacks |
|--------|--------|
|        |        |

| Supplements | Medication |
|-------------|------------|
|             |            |

Date ............................................................................................................

Sleep quality and duration ....................................................................

Stress levels     1    2    3    4    5    6    7    8    9    10

| Time | Systolic | Diastolic | Heart Rate |
|------|----------|-----------|------------|
|      |          |           |            |
|      |          |           |            |
|      |          |           |            |
|      |          |           |            |
|      |          |           |            |

Exercise and daily activities      Water Intake ⬜⬜⬜⬜⬜⬜⬜

..............................................................

..............................................................

..............................................................

..............................................................

..............................................................

..............................................................

..............................................................

..............................................................

..............................................................

..............................................................

..............................................................

..............................................................

..............................................................

| Breakfast | Lunch |
|-----------|-------|
|           |       |

| Dinner | Snacks |
|--------|--------|
|        |        |

| Supplements | Medication |
|-------------|------------|
|             |            |

Date ................................................................................................

Sleep quality and duration ...............................................................

Stress levels    1   2   3   4   5   6   7   8   9   10

| Time | Systolic | Diastolic | Heart Rate |
|---|---|---|---|
|  |  |  |  |
|  |  |  |  |
|  |  |  |  |
|  |  |  |  |
|  |  |  |  |

Exercise and daily activities     Water Intake

..............................................................

..............................................................

..............................................................

..............................................................

..............................................................

..............................................................

..............................................................

..............................................................

..............................................................

..............................................................

..............................................................

..............................................................

..............................................................

..............................................................

..............................................................

| Breakfast | Lunch |
|---|---|
|  |  |

| Dinner | Snacks |
|---|---|
|  |  |

| Supplements | Medication |
|---|---|
|  |  |

Date .................................................................................................

Sleep quality and duration ...........................................................

Stress levels      1    2    3    4    5    6    7    8    9    10

| Time | Systolic | Diastolic | Heart Rate |
|---|---|---|---|
| | | | |
| | | | |
| | | | |
| | | | |
| | | | |

Exercise and daily activities        Water Intake

| Breakfast | Lunch |
|---|---|
| | |
| Dinner | Snacks |
| | |
| Supplements | Medication |
| | |

Date ..................................................................................................................

Sleep quality and duration .........................................................................

Stress levels     1   2   3   4   5   6   7   8   9   10

| Time | Systolic | Diastolic | Heart Rate |
|---|---|---|---|
|  |  |  |  |
|  |  |  |  |
|  |  |  |  |
|  |  |  |  |
|  |  |  |  |

Exercise and daily activities        Water Intake

..........................................................

..........................................................

..........................................................

..........................................................

..........................................................

..........................................................

..........................................................

..........................................................

..........................................................

..........................................................

..........................................................

..........................................................

..........................................................

..........................................................

| Breakfast | Lunch |
|---|---|
|  |  |

| Dinner | Snacks |
|---|---|
|  |  |

| Supplements | Medication |
|---|---|
|  |  |

Date .............................................................................................................

Sleep quality and duration ..................................................................................

Stress levels      1    2    3    4    5    6    7    8    9    10

| Time | Systolic | Diastolic | Heart Rate |
|---|---|---|---|
|  |  |  |  |
|  |  |  |  |
|  |  |  |  |
|  |  |  |  |
|  |  |  |  |

Exercise and daily activities      Water Intake ☐☐☐☐☐☐☐☐

| Breakfast | Lunch |
|---|---|
|  |  |

| Dinner | Snacks |
|---|---|
|  |  |

| Supplements | Medication |
|---|---|
|  |  |

Date .................................................................................................................................

Sleep quality and duration ..............................................................................

Stress levels      1    2    3    4    5    6    7    8    9    10

| Time | Systolic | Diastolic | Heart Rate |
|---|---|---|---|
|  |  |  |  |
|  |  |  |  |
|  |  |  |  |
|  |  |  |  |
|  |  |  |  |

Exercise and daily activities      Water Intake

| Breakfast | Lunch |
|---|---|
|  |  |
| Dinner | Snacks |
|  |  |
| Supplements | Medication |
|  |  |

Date ...........................................................................................................

Sleep quality and duration ....................................................................

Stress levels      1    2    3    4    5    6    7    8    9    10

| Time | Systolic | Diastolic | Heart Rate |
|------|----------|-----------|------------|
|      |          |           |            |
|      |          |           |            |
|      |          |           |            |
|      |          |           |            |
|      |          |           |            |

Exercise and daily activities      Water Intake

...................................................
...................................................
...................................................
...................................................
...................................................
...................................................
...................................................
...................................................
...................................................
...................................................
...................................................
...................................................
...................................................
...................................................
...................................................

| Breakfast | Lunch |
|-----------|-------|
|           |       |

| Dinner | Snacks |
|--------|--------|
|        |        |

| Supplements | Medication |
|-------------|------------|
|             |            |

Date .................................................................................

Sleep quality and duration ...........................................

Stress levels      1    2    3    4    5    6    7    8    9    10

| Time | Systolic | Diastolic | Heart Rate |
|---|---|---|---|
|  |  |  |  |
|  |  |  |  |
|  |  |  |  |
|  |  |  |  |
|  |  |  |  |

Exercise and daily activities      Water Intake

| Breakfast | Lunch |
|---|---|
|  |  |

| Dinner | Snacks |
|---|---|
|  |  |

| Supplements | Medication |
|---|---|
|  |  |

Date .......................................................................................................

Sleep quality and duration ...................................................................

Stress levels      1    2    3    4    5    6    7    8    9    10

| Time | Systolic | Diastolic | Heart Rate |
|---|---|---|---|
|  |  |  |  |
|  |  |  |  |
|  |  |  |  |
|  |  |  |  |
|  |  |  |  |

Exercise and daily activities      Water Intake

..................................................................

..................................................................

..................................................................

..................................................................

..................................................................

..................................................................

..................................................................

..................................................................

..................................................................

..................................................................

..................................................................

..................................................................

..................................................................

..................................................................

| Breakfast | Lunch |
|---|---|
|  |  |
| Dinner | Snacks |
|  |  |
| Supplements | Medication |
|  |  |

Date .............................................................................................................

Sleep quality and duration ...................................................................

Stress levels      1    2    3    4    5    6    7    8    9    10

| Time | Systolic | Diastolic | Heart Rate |
|------|----------|-----------|------------|
|      |          |           |            |
|      |          |           |            |
|      |          |           |            |
|      |          |           |            |
|      |          |           |            |

**Exercise and daily activities**

**Water Intake**

...........................................................

...........................................................

...........................................................

...........................................................

...........................................................

...........................................................

...........................................................

...........................................................

...........................................................

...........................................................

...........................................................

...........................................................

...........................................................

...........................................................

...........................................................

| Breakfast | Lunch |
|-----------|-------|
|           |       |

| Dinner | Snacks |
|--------|--------|
|        |        |

| Supplements | Medication |
|-------------|------------|
|             |            |

Date ............................................................................................................

Sleep quality and duration .............................................................................

Stress levels      1    2    3    4    5    6    7    8    9    10

| Time | Systolic | Diastolic | Heart Rate |
|------|----------|-----------|------------|
|      |          |           |            |
|      |          |           |            |
|      |          |           |            |
|      |          |           |            |
|      |          |           |            |

Exercise and daily activities      Water Intake

| Breakfast | Lunch |
|-----------|-------|
|           |       |

| Dinner | Snacks |
|--------|--------|
|        |        |

| Supplements | Medication |
|-------------|------------|
|             |            |

Date .............................................................................................................

Sleep quality and duration .......................................................................

Stress levels      1    2    3    4    5    6    7    8    9    10

| Time | Systolic | Diastolic | Heart Rate |
|---|---|---|---|
|  |  |  |  |
|  |  |  |  |
|  |  |  |  |
|  |  |  |  |
|  |  |  |  |

**Exercise and daily activities**　　　　Water Intake ⬜⬜⬜⬜⬜⬜⬜

| Breakfast | Lunch |
|---|---|
|  |  |

| Dinner | Snacks |
|---|---|
|  |  |

| Supplements | Medication |
|---|---|
|  |  |

Date .........................................................................................................

Sleep quality and duration ...........................................................................

Stress levels     1    2    3    4    5    6    7    8    9    10

| Time | Systolic | Diastolic | Heart Rate |
|---|---|---|---|
|  |  |  |  |
|  |  |  |  |
|  |  |  |  |
|  |  |  |  |
|  |  |  |  |

**Exercise and daily activities**       Water Intake

......................................................

......................................................

......................................................

......................................................

......................................................

......................................................

......................................................

......................................................

......................................................

......................................................

......................................................

......................................................

......................................................

......................................................

| Breakfast | Lunch |
|---|---|
|  |  |

| Dinner | Snacks |
|---|---|
|  |  |

| Supplements | Medication |
|---|---|
|  |  |

Date .................................................................................................................

Sleep quality and duration ...........................................................................

Stress levels      1    2    3    4    5    6    7    8    9    10

| Time | Systolic | Diastolic | Heart Rate |
|------|----------|-----------|------------|
|      |          |           |            |
|      |          |           |            |
|      |          |           |            |
|      |          |           |            |
|      |          |           |            |

Exercise and daily activities      Water Intake

| Breakfast | Lunch |
|-----------|-------|
|           |       |

| Dinner | Snacks |
|--------|--------|
|        |        |

| Supplements | Medication |
|-------------|------------|
|             |            |

Date .................................................................................................

Sleep quality and duration .................................................................

Stress levels     1    2    3    4    5    6    7    8    9    10

| Time | Systolic | Diastolic | Heart Rate |
|------|----------|-----------|------------|
|      |          |           |            |
|      |          |           |            |
|      |          |           |            |
|      |          |           |            |
|      |          |           |            |

Exercise and daily activities      Water Intake ⬜⬜⬜⬜⬜⬜⬜

| Breakfast | Lunch |
|-----------|-------|
|           |       |

| Dinner | Snacks |
|--------|--------|
|        |        |

| Supplements | Medication |
|-------------|------------|
|             |            |

Date .................................................................................................

Sleep quality and duration ...........................................................

Stress levels      1   2   3   4   5   6   7   8   9   10

| Time | Systolic | Diastolic | Heart Rate |
|---|---|---|---|
|  |  |  |  |
|  |  |  |  |
|  |  |  |  |
|  |  |  |  |
|  |  |  |  |

Exercise and daily activities      Water Intake

..............................................................

..............................................................

..............................................................

..............................................................

..............................................................

..............................................................

..............................................................

..............................................................

..............................................................

..............................................................

..............................................................

..............................................................

..............................................................

..............................................................

| Breakfast | Lunch |
|---|---|
|  |  |

| Dinner | Snacks |
|---|---|
|  |  |

| Supplements | Medication |
|---|---|
|  |  |

Date ..............................................................................

Sleep quality and duration ...............................................

Stress levels      1    2    3    4    5    6    7    8    9    10

| Time | Systolic | Diastolic | Heart Rate |
|---|---|---|---|
|  |  |  |  |
|  |  |  |  |
|  |  |  |  |
|  |  |  |  |
|  |  |  |  |

Exercise and daily activities      Water Intake ▢▢▢▢▢▢▢

......................................................

......................................................

......................................................

......................................................

......................................................

......................................................

......................................................

......................................................

......................................................

......................................................

......................................................

......................................................

......................................................

| Breakfast | Lunch |
|---|---|
|  |  |

| Dinner | Snacks |
|---|---|
|  |  |

| Supplements | Medication |
|---|---|
|  |  |

Date .............................................................................................................

Sleep quality and duration ........................................................................

Stress levels      1    2    3    4    5    6    7    8    9    10

| Time | Systolic | Diastolic | Heart Rate |
|---|---|---|---|
|  |  |  |  |
|  |  |  |  |
|  |  |  |  |
|  |  |  |  |
|  |  |  |  |

Exercise and daily activities      Water Intake

.................................................................
.................................................................
.................................................................
.................................................................
.................................................................
.................................................................
.................................................................
.................................................................
.................................................................
.................................................................
.................................................................
.................................................................
.................................................................
.................................................................
.................................................................
.................................................................

| Breakfast | Lunch |
|---|---|
|  |  |

| Dinner | Snacks |
|---|---|
|  |  |

| Supplements | Medication |
|---|---|
|  |  |

Date .............................................................................................

Sleep quality and duration .......................................................

Stress levels     1   2   3   4   5   6   7   8   9   10

| Time | Systolic | Diastolic | Heart Rate |
|------|----------|-----------|------------|
|      |          |           |            |
|      |          |           |            |
|      |          |           |            |
|      |          |           |            |

**Exercise and daily activities**     **Water Intake**

| Breakfast | Lunch |
|-----------|-------|
|           |       |

| Dinner | Snacks |
|--------|--------|
|        |        |

| Supplements | Medication |
|-------------|------------|
|             |            |

Date ..............................................................................................

Sleep quality and duration ...................................................................

Stress levels       1    2    3    4    5    6    7    8    9    10

| Time | Systolic | Diastolic | Heart Rate |
|------|----------|-----------|------------|
|      |          |           |            |
|      |          |           |            |
|      |          |           |            |
|      |          |           |            |
|      |          |           |            |

Exercise and daily activities          Water Intake ⬚⬚⬚⬚⬚⬚⬚⬚

..............................................................

..............................................................

..............................................................

..............................................................

..............................................................

..............................................................

..............................................................

..............................................................

..............................................................

..............................................................

..............................................................

..............................................................

..............................................................

..............................................................

..............................................................

| Breakfast | Lunch |
|-----------|-------|
|           |       |

| Dinner | Snacks |
|--------|--------|
|        |        |

| Supplements | Medication |
|-------------|------------|
|             |            |

Date .................................................................................................

Sleep quality and duration .........................................................

Stress levels      1    2    3    4    5    6    7    8    9    10

| Time | Systolic | Diastolic | Heart Rate |
|---|---|---|---|
|  |  |  |  |
|  |  |  |  |
|  |  |  |  |
|  |  |  |  |
|  |  |  |  |

Exercise and daily activities       Water Intake

| Breakfast | Lunch |
|---|---|
|  |  |
| Dinner | Snacks |
|  |  |
| Supplements | Medication |
|  |  |

Date ................................................................................

Sleep quality and duration ................................................

Stress levels     1   2   3   4   5   6   7   8   9   10

| Time | Systolic | Diastolic | Heart Rate |
|------|----------|-----------|------------|
|      |          |           |            |
|      |          |           |            |
|      |          |           |            |
|      |          |           |            |
|      |          |           |            |

Exercise and daily activities     Water Intake

..............................................

..............................................

..............................................

..............................................

..............................................

..............................................

..............................................

..............................................

..............................................

..............................................

..............................................

..............................................

..............................................

..............................................

..............................................

| Breakfast | Lunch |
|-----------|-------|
|           |       |

| Dinner | Snacks |
|--------|--------|
|        |        |

| Supplements | Medication |
|-------------|------------|
|             |            |

Date .................................................................................

Sleep quality and duration ...........................................................

Stress levels      1    2    3    4    5    6    7    8    9    10

| Time | Systolic | Diastolic | Heart Rate |
|---|---|---|---|
|  |  |  |  |
|  |  |  |  |
|  |  |  |  |
|  |  |  |  |
|  |  |  |  |

**Exercise and daily activities**      **Water Intake**

| Breakfast | Lunch |
|---|---|
|  |  |

| Dinner | Snacks |
|---|---|
|  |  |

| Supplements | Medication |
|---|---|
|  |  |

Date .............................................................................................................

Sleep quality and duration .........................................................................

Stress levels     1    2    3    4    5    6    7    8    9    10

| Time | Systolic | Diastolic | Heart Rate |
|------|----------|-----------|------------|
|      |          |           |            |
|      |          |           |            |
|      |          |           |            |
|      |          |           |            |
|      |          |           |            |

**Exercise and daily activities**       **Water Intake** ☐ ☐ ☐ ☐ ☐ ☐

..............................................................

..............................................................

..............................................................

..............................................................

..............................................................

..............................................................

..............................................................

..............................................................

..............................................................

..............................................................

..............................................................

..............................................................

..............................................................

..............................................................

..............................................................

| Breakfast | Lunch |
|-----------|-------|
|           |       |

| Dinner | Snacks |
|--------|--------|
|        |        |

| Supplements | Medication |
|-------------|------------|
|             |            |

Date .......................................................................

Sleep quality and duration .......................................................

Stress levels     1    2    3    4    5    6    7    8    9    10

| Time | Systolic | Diastolic | Heart Rate |
|------|----------|-----------|------------|
|      |          |           |            |
|      |          |           |            |
|      |          |           |            |
|      |          |           |            |
|      |          |           |            |

Exercise and daily activities      Water Intake ☐☐☐☐☐☐☐

| Breakfast | Lunch |
|-----------|-------|
|           |       |

| Dinner | Snacks |
|--------|--------|
|        |        |

| Supplements | Medication |
|-------------|------------|
|             |            |

Date .........................................................................................................

Sleep quality and duration ...............................................................

Stress levels      1    2    3    4    5    6    7    8    9    10

| Time | Systolic | Diastolic | Heart Rate |
|------|----------|-----------|------------|
|      |          |           |            |
|      |          |           |            |
|      |          |           |            |
|      |          |           |            |
|      |          |           |            |

Exercise and daily activities      Water Intake

| Breakfast | Lunch |
|-----------|-------|
|           |       |

| Dinner | Snacks |
|--------|--------|
|        |        |

| Supplements | Medication |
|-------------|------------|
|             |            |

Date .................................................................................................

Sleep quality and duration ....................................................................

Stress levels     1   2   3   4   5   6   7   8   9   10

| Time | Systolic | Diastolic | Heart Rate |
|------|----------|-----------|------------|
|      |          |           |            |
|      |          |           |            |
|      |          |           |            |
|      |          |           |            |
|      |          |           |            |

Exercise and daily activities       Water Intake

| Breakfast | Lunch |
|-----------|-------|
|           |       |

| Dinner | Snacks |
|--------|--------|
|        |        |

| Supplements | Medication |
|-------------|------------|
|             |            |

Date ........................................................................................................................

Sleep quality and duration ...........................................................................

Stress levels     1    2    3    4    5    6    7    8    9    10

| Time | Systolic | Diastolic | Heart Rate |
|------|----------|-----------|------------|
|      |          |           |            |
|      |          |           |            |
|      |          |           |            |
|      |          |           |            |
|      |          |           |            |

Exercise and daily activities      Water Intake

....................................................

....................................................

....................................................

....................................................

....................................................

....................................................

....................................................

....................................................

....................................................

....................................................

....................................................

....................................................

....................................................

....................................................

....................................................

| Breakfast | Lunch |
|-----------|-------|
|           |       |

| Dinner | Snacks |
|--------|--------|
|        |        |

| Supplements | Medication |
|-------------|------------|
|             |            |

Date .................................................................................................

Sleep quality and duration ...................................................................

Stress levels     1    2    3    4    5    6    7    8    9    10

| Time | Systolic | Diastolic | Heart Rate |
|---|---|---|---|
|  |  |  |  |
|  |  |  |  |
|  |  |  |  |
|  |  |  |  |
|  |  |  |  |

Exercise and daily activities       Water Intake

| Breakfast | Lunch |
|---|---|
|  |  |

| Dinner | Snacks |
|---|---|
|  |  |

| Supplements | Medication |
|---|---|
|  |  |

Date  ................................................................................................................

Sleep quality and duration  ...................................................................................

Stress levels       1    2    3    4    5    6    7    8    9    10

| Time | Systolic | Diastolic | Heart Rate |
|---|---|---|---|
|  |  |  |  |
|  |  |  |  |
|  |  |  |  |
|  |  |  |  |
|  |  |  |  |

Exercise and daily activities        Water Intake

| Breakfast | Lunch |
|---|---|
|  |  |
| Dinner | Snacks |
|  |  |
| Supplements | Medication |
|  |  |

Date ...................................................................................................

Sleep quality and duration ...................................................................

Stress levels          1    2    3    4    5    6    7    8    9    10

| Time | Systolic | Diastolic | Heart Rate |
|---|---|---|---|
|  |  |  |  |
|  |  |  |  |
|  |  |  |  |
|  |  |  |  |
|  |  |  |  |

Exercise and daily activities          Water Intake

..................................................

..................................................

..................................................

..................................................

..................................................

..................................................

..................................................

..................................................

..................................................

..................................................

..................................................

..................................................

..................................................

| Breakfast | Lunch |
|---|---|
|  |  |
| Dinner | Snacks |
|  |  |
| Supplements | Medication |
|  |  |

Date .........................................................................................................

Sleep quality and duration ...............................................................

Stress levels     1    2    3    4    5    6    7    8    9    10

| Time | Systolic | Diastolic | Heart Rate |
|---|---|---|---|
|  |  |  |  |
|  |  |  |  |
|  |  |  |  |
|  |  |  |  |
|  |  |  |  |

Exercise and daily activities      Water Intake

| Breakfast | Lunch |
|---|---|
|  |  |

| Dinner | Snacks |
|---|---|
|  |  |

| Supplements | Medication |
|---|---|
|  |  |

Date .....................................................................................

Sleep quality and duration ...............................................

Stress levels        1    2    3    4    5    6    7    8    9    10

| Time | Systolic | Diastolic | Heart Rate |
|------|----------|-----------|------------|
|      |          |           |            |
|      |          |           |            |
|      |          |           |            |
|      |          |           |            |
|      |          |           |            |

Exercise and daily activities          Water Intake

...............................................

...............................................

...............................................

...............................................

...............................................

...............................................

...............................................

...............................................

...............................................

...............................................

...............................................

...............................................

...............................................

...............................................

| Breakfast | Lunch |
|-----------|-------|
|           |       |

| Dinner | Snacks |
|--------|--------|
|        |        |

| Supplements | Medication |
|-------------|------------|
|             |            |

Date ...........................................................................................

Sleep quality and duration ...............................................................

Stress levels     1    2    3    4    5    6    7    8    9    10

| Time | Systolic | Diastolic | Heart Rate |
|---|---|---|---|
|  |  |  |  |
|  |  |  |  |
|  |  |  |  |
|  |  |  |  |
|  |  |  |  |

**Exercise and daily activities**

     Water Intake ☐☐☐☐☐☐☐

| Breakfast | Lunch |
|---|---|
|  |  |

| Dinner | Snacks |
|---|---|
|  |  |

| Supplements | Medication |
|---|---|
|  |  |

Date .................................................................................

Sleep quality and duration .................................................

Stress levels     1   2   3   4   5   6   7   8   9   10

| Time | Systolic | Diastolic | Heart Rate |
|------|----------|-----------|------------|
|      |          |           |            |
|      |          |           |            |
|      |          |           |            |
|      |          |           |            |
|      |          |           |            |

Exercise and daily activities      Water Intake

| Breakfast | Lunch |
|-----------|-------|
|           |       |

| Dinner | Snacks |
|--------|--------|
|        |        |

| Supplements | Medication |
|-------------|------------|
|             |            |

Date .................................................................................................

Sleep quality and duration ...........................................................

Stress levels      1   2   3   4   5   6   7   8   9   10

| Time | Systolic | Diastolic | Heart Rate |
|---|---|---|---|
|  |  |  |  |
|  |  |  |  |
|  |  |  |  |
|  |  |  |  |
|  |  |  |  |

Exercise and daily activities      Water Intake

| Breakfast | Lunch |
|---|---|
|  |  |

| Dinner | Snacks |
|---|---|
|  |  |

| Supplements | Medication |
|---|---|
|  |  |

Date ...........................................................................................

Sleep quality and duration .................................................................

Stress levels     1   2   3   4   5   6   7   8   9   10

| Time | Systolic | Diastolic | Heart Rate |
|---|---|---|---|
|  |  |  |  |
|  |  |  |  |
|  |  |  |  |
|  |  |  |  |
|  |  |  |  |

Exercise and daily activities       Water Intake

| Breakfast | Lunch |
|---|---|
|  |  |
| Dinner | Snacks |
|  |  |
| Supplements | Medication |
|  |  |

Date ..............................................................................................................

Sleep quality and duration ............................................................................

Stress levels      1    2    3    4    5    6    7    8    9    10

| Time | Systolic | Diastolic | Heart Rate |
|---|---|---|---|
|  |  |  |  |
|  |  |  |  |
|  |  |  |  |
|  |  |  |  |
|  |  |  |  |

Exercise and daily activities        Water Intake

..............................................................

..............................................................

..............................................................

..............................................................

..............................................................

..............................................................

..............................................................

..............................................................

..............................................................

..............................................................

..............................................................

..............................................................

..............................................................

..............................................................

..............................................................

| Breakfast | Lunch |
|---|---|
|  |  |
| Dinner | Snacks |
|  |  |
| Supplements | Medication |
|  |  |

Date .........................................................................................

Sleep quality and duration ...........................................................

Stress levels     1    2    3    4    5    6    7    8    9    10

| Time | Systolic | Diastolic | Heart Rate |
|---|---|---|---|
|  |  |  |  |
|  |  |  |  |
|  |  |  |  |
|  |  |  |  |
|  |  |  |  |

Exercise and daily activities    Water Intake

| Breakfast | Lunch |
|---|---|
|  |  |
| Dinner | Snacks |
|  |  |
| Supplements | Medication |
|  |  |

Date ...........................................................................................................................

Sleep quality and duration ...........................................................................

Stress levels     1    2    3    4    5    6    7    8    9    10

| Time | Systolic | Diastolic | Heart Rate |
|---|---|---|---|
|  |  |  |  |
|  |  |  |  |
|  |  |  |  |
|  |  |  |  |
|  |  |  |  |

Exercise and daily activities      Water Intake ⬜⬜⬜⬜⬜⬜⬜

..................................................................
..................................................................
..................................................................
..................................................................
..................................................................
..................................................................
..................................................................
..................................................................
..................................................................
..................................................................
..................................................................
..................................................................
..................................................................
..................................................................

| Breakfast | Lunch |
|---|---|
|  |  |

| Dinner | Snacks |
|---|---|
|  |  |

| Supplements | Medication |
|---|---|
|  |  |

Date .........................................................................................................................

Sleep quality and duration .........................................................................

Stress levels      1    2    3    4    5    6    7    8    9    10

| Time | Systolic | Diastolic | Heart Rate |
|------|----------|-----------|------------|
|      |          |           |            |
|      |          |           |            |
|      |          |           |            |
|      |          |           |            |
|      |          |           |            |

Exercise and daily activities      Water Intake

| Breakfast | Lunch |
|-----------|-------|
|           |       |

| Dinner | Snacks |
|--------|--------|
|        |        |

| Supplements | Medication |
|-------------|------------|
|             |            |

Date ...........................................................................................................................

Sleep quality and duration ...........................................................................................

Stress levels      1    2    3    4    5    6    7    8    9    10

| Time | Systolic | Diastolic | Heart Rate |
|---|---|---|---|
|  |  |  |  |
|  |  |  |  |
|  |  |  |  |
|  |  |  |  |
|  |  |  |  |

Exercise and daily activities       Water Intake

....................................................

....................................................

....................................................

....................................................

....................................................

....................................................

....................................................

....................................................

....................................................

....................................................

....................................................

....................................................

....................................................

....................................................

....................................................

| Breakfast | Lunch |
|---|---|
|  |  |
| Dinner | Snacks |
|  |  |
| Supplements | Medication |
|  |  |

Date ........................................................................................................

Sleep quality and duration ...............................................................

Stress levels     1    2    3    4    5    6    7    8    9    10

| Time | Systolic | Diastolic | Heart Rate |
|---|---|---|---|
|  |  |  |  |
|  |  |  |  |
|  |  |  |  |
|  |  |  |  |
|  |  |  |  |

Exercise and daily activities     Water Intake ☐☐☐☐☐☐☐☐

| Breakfast | Lunch |
|---|---|
|  |  |
| Dinner | Snacks |
|  |  |
| Supplements | Medication |
|  |  |

Date ...................................................................................................

Sleep quality and duration .................................................................

Stress levels     1   2   3   4   5   6   7   8   9   10

| Time | Systolic | Diastolic | Heart Rate |
|------|----------|-----------|------------|
|      |          |           |            |
|      |          |           |            |
|      |          |           |            |
|      |          |           |            |
|      |          |           |            |

Exercise and daily activities      Water Intake

| Breakfast | Lunch |
|-----------|-------|
|           |       |

| Dinner | Snacks |
|--------|--------|
|        |        |

| Supplements | Medication |
|-------------|------------|
|             |            |

Date .................................................................................................................

Sleep quality and duration ...........................................................................

Stress levels     1    2    3    4    5    6    7    8    9    10

| Time | Systolic | Diastolic | Heart Rate |
|---|---|---|---|
| | | | |
| | | | |
| | | | |
| | | | |
| | | | |

Exercise and daily activities       Water Intake

| Breakfast | Lunch |
|---|---|
| | |
| **Dinner** | **Snacks** |
| | |
| **Supplements** | **Medication** |
| | |

Date .............................................................................

Sleep quality and duration ...........................................................

Stress levels      1   2   3   4   5   6   7   8   9   10

| Time | Systolic | Diastolic | Heart Rate |
|---|---|---|---|
|  |  |  |  |
|  |  |  |  |
|  |  |  |  |
|  |  |  |  |
|  |  |  |  |

Exercise and daily activities

Water Intake

| Breakfast | Lunch |
|---|---|
|  |  |

| Dinner | Snacks |
|---|---|
|  |  |

| Supplements | Medication |
|---|---|
|  |  |

Date  ...........................................................................................

Sleep quality and duration  ...............................................................

Stress levels     1    2    3    4    5    6    7    8    9    10

| Time | Systolic | Diastolic | Heart Rate |
|---|---|---|---|
|  |  |  |  |
|  |  |  |  |
|  |  |  |  |
|  |  |  |  |
|  |  |  |  |

Exercise and daily activities       Water Intake

| Breakfast | Lunch |
|---|---|
|  |  |
| Dinner | Snacks |
|  |  |
| Supplements | Medication |
|  |  |

Date .................................................................................................

Sleep quality and duration .......................................................

Stress levels     1   2   3   4   5   6   7   8   9   10

| Time | Systolic | Diastolic | Heart Rate |
|------|----------|-----------|------------|
|      |          |           |            |
|      |          |           |            |
|      |          |           |            |
|      |          |           |            |
|      |          |           |            |

Exercise and daily activities      Water Intake

| Breakfast | Lunch |
|-----------|-------|
|           |       |

| Dinner | Snacks |
|--------|--------|
|        |        |

| Supplements | Medication |
|-------------|------------|
|             |            |

Date ........................................................................................

Sleep quality and duration ...........................................................

Stress levels     1   2   3   4   5   6   7   8   9   10

| Time | Systolic | Diastolic | Heart Rate |
|------|----------|-----------|------------|
|      |          |           |            |
|      |          |           |            |
|      |          |           |            |
|      |          |           |            |
|      |          |           |            |

Exercise and daily activities     Water Intake ⬜⬜⬜⬜⬜⬜⬜

..............................................

..............................................

..............................................

..............................................

..............................................

..............................................

..............................................

..............................................

..............................................

..............................................

..............................................

..............................................

..............................................

| Breakfast | Lunch |
|-----------|-------|
|           |       |

| Dinner | Snacks |
|--------|--------|
|        |        |

| Supplements | Medication |
|-------------|------------|
|             |            |

Date  .............................................................................................................

Sleep quality and duration  ....................................................................

Stress levels       1    2    3    4    5    6    7    8    9    10

| Time | Systolic | Diastolic | Heart Rate |
|---|---|---|---|
|  |  |  |  |
|  |  |  |  |
|  |  |  |  |
|  |  |  |  |

Exercise and daily activities        Water Intake

| Breakfast | Lunch |
|---|---|
|  |  |
| Dinner | Snacks |
|  |  |
| Supplements | Medication |
|  |  |

Date ..........................................................................................

Sleep quality and duration ..............................................................

Stress levels        1    2    3    4    5    6    7    8    9    10

| Time | Systolic | Diastolic | Heart Rate |
|---|---|---|---|
|  |  |  |  |
|  |  |  |  |
|  |  |  |  |
|  |  |  |  |
|  |  |  |  |

Exercise and daily activities          Water Intake

..................................................

..................................................

..................................................

..................................................

..................................................

..................................................

..................................................

..................................................

..................................................

..................................................

..................................................

..................................................

..................................................

| Breakfast | Lunch |
|---|---|
|  |  |
| Dinner | Snacks |
|  |  |
| Supplements | Medication |
|  |  |

Date .................................................................................................

Sleep quality and duration .......................................................................

Stress levels     1    2    3    4    5    6    7    8    9    10

| Time | Systolic | Diastolic | Heart Rate |
|---|---|---|---|
|  |  |  |  |
|  |  |  |  |
|  |  |  |  |
|  |  |  |  |
|  |  |  |  |

Exercise and daily activities      Water Intake

| Breakfast | Lunch |
|---|---|
|  |  |
| Dinner | Snacks |
|  |  |
| Supplements | Medication |
|  |  |

Date  ...............................................................................

Sleep quality and duration  ...............................................................................

Stress levels     1   2   3   4   5   6   7   8   9   10

| Time | Systolic | Diastolic | Heart Rate |
|---|---|---|---|
|  |  |  |  |
|  |  |  |  |
|  |  |  |  |
|  |  |  |  |
|  |  |  |  |

Exercise and daily activities       Water Intake

....................................................

....................................................

....................................................

....................................................

....................................................

....................................................

....................................................

....................................................

....................................................

....................................................

....................................................

....................................................

....................................................

....................................................

| Breakfast | Lunch |
|---|---|
|  |  |

| Dinner | Snacks |
|---|---|
|  |  |

| Supplements | Medication |
|---|---|
|  |  |

Date ........................................................................................

Sleep quality and duration ...................................................

Stress levels     1   2   3   4   5   6   7   8   9   10

| Time | Systolic | Diastolic | Heart Rate |
|------|----------|-----------|------------|
|      |          |           |            |
|      |          |           |            |
|      |          |           |            |
|      |          |           |            |
|      |          |           |            |

Exercise and daily activities      Water Intake

| Breakfast | Lunch |
|-----------|-------|
|           |       |

| Dinner | Snacks |
|--------|--------|
|        |        |

| Supplements | Medication |
|-------------|------------|
|             |            |

Date ....................................................................................................................

Sleep quality and duration .................................................................................

Stress levels      1    2    3    4    5    6    7    8    9    10

| Time | Systolic | Diastolic | Heart Rate |
|------|----------|-----------|------------|
|      |          |           |            |
|      |          |           |            |
|      |          |           |            |
|      |          |           |            |
|      |          |           |            |

Exercise and daily activities        Water Intake

....................................................................
....................................................................
....................................................................
....................................................................
....................................................................
....................................................................
....................................................................
....................................................................
....................................................................
....................................................................
....................................................................
....................................................................
....................................................................
....................................................................

| Breakfast | Lunch |
|-----------|-------|
|           |       |

| Dinner | Snacks |
|--------|--------|
|        |        |

| Supplements | Medication |
|-------------|------------|
|             |            |

Date .................................................................................................

Sleep quality and duration  ...............................................................

Stress levels      1    2    3    4    5    6    7    8    9    10

| Time | Systolic | Diastolic | Heart Rate |
|------|----------|-----------|------------|
|      |          |           |            |
|      |          |           |            |
|      |          |           |            |
|      |          |           |            |
|      |          |           |            |

Exercise and daily activities          Water Intake

.................................................

.................................................

.................................................

.................................................

.................................................

.................................................

.................................................

.................................................

.................................................

.................................................

.................................................

.................................................

.................................................

.................................................

| Breakfast | Lunch |
|-----------|-------|
|           |       |

| Dinner | Snacks |
|--------|--------|
|        |        |

| Supplements | Medication |
|-------------|------------|
|             |            |

Date ............................................................................................................

Sleep quality and duration ...........................................................................

Stress levels     1    2    3    4    5    6    7    8    9    10

| Time | Systolic | Diastolic | Heart Rate |
|------|----------|-----------|------------|
|      |          |           |            |
|      |          |           |            |
|      |          |           |            |
|      |          |           |            |
|      |          |           |            |

Exercise and daily activities      Water Intake

| Breakfast | Lunch |
|-----------|-------|
|           |       |

| Dinner | Snacks |
|--------|--------|
|        |        |

| Supplements | Medication |
|-------------|------------|
|             |            |

Date .................................................................................................................

Sleep quality and duration ...........................................................................

Stress levels      1    2    3    4    5    6    7    8    9    10

| Time | Systolic | Diastolic | Heart Rate |
|------|----------|-----------|------------|
|      |          |           |            |
|      |          |           |            |
|      |          |           |            |
|      |          |           |            |
|      |          |           |            |

Exercise and daily activities      Water Intake

| Breakfast | Lunch |
|-----------|-------|
|           |       |
| Dinner | Snacks |
|        |        |
| Supplements | Medication |
|             |            |

Date ............................................................................................................

Sleep quality and duration ...........................................................................

Stress levels     1    2    3    4    5    6    7    8    9    10

| Time | Systolic | Diastolic | Heart Rate |
|---|---|---|---|
|  |  |  |  |
|  |  |  |  |
|  |  |  |  |
|  |  |  |  |
|  |  |  |  |

Exercise and daily activities      Water Intake

| Breakfast | Lunch |
|---|---|
|  |  |
| Dinner | Snacks |
|  |  |
| Supplements | Medication |
|  |  |

Date ...................................................................................................

Sleep quality and duration ...........................................................

Stress levels     1    2    3    4    5    6    7    8    9    10

| Time | Systolic | Diastolic | Heart Rate |
|---|---|---|---|
|  |  |  |  |
|  |  |  |  |
|  |  |  |  |
|  |  |  |  |
|  |  |  |  |

**Exercise and daily activities**

Water Intake ☐ ☐ ☐ ☐ ☐ ☐ ☐

..................................................................

..................................................................

..................................................................

..................................................................

..................................................................

..................................................................

..................................................................

..................................................................

..................................................................

..................................................................

..................................................................

..................................................................

..................................................................

..................................................................

| Breakfast | Lunch |
|---|---|
|  |  |

| Dinner | Snacks |
|---|---|
|  |  |

| Supplements | Medication |
|---|---|
|  |  |

Date .............................................................................................................

Sleep quality and duration ...........................................................................

Stress levels      1    2    3    4    5    6    7    8    9    10

| Time | Systolic | Diastolic | Heart Rate |
|---|---|---|---|
|  |  |  |  |
|  |  |  |  |
|  |  |  |  |
|  |  |  |  |
|  |  |  |  |

Exercise and daily activities      Water Intake

| Breakfast | Lunch |
|---|---|
|  |  |
| Dinner | Snacks |
|  |  |
| Supplements | Medication |
|  |  |

Date .............................................................................................................

Sleep quality and duration ...................................................................

Stress levels     1    2    3    4    5    6    7    8    9    10

| Time | Systolic | Diastolic | Heart Rate |
|------|----------|-----------|------------|
|      |          |           |            |
|      |          |           |            |
|      |          |           |            |
|      |          |           |            |
|      |          |           |            |

Exercise and daily activities      Water Intake

| Breakfast | Lunch |
|-----------|-------|
|           |       |

| Dinner | Snacks |
|--------|--------|
|        |        |

| Supplements | Medication |
|-------------|------------|
|             |            |

Date ...........................................................................................................

Sleep quality and duration ...........................................................................

Stress levels     1   2   3   4   5   6   7   8   9   10

| Time | Systolic | Diastolic | Heart Rate |
|------|----------|-----------|------------|
|      |          |           |            |
|      |          |           |            |
|      |          |           |            |
|      |          |           |            |
|      |          |           |            |

Exercise and daily activities     Water Intake

| Breakfast | Lunch |
|-----------|-------|
|           |       |

| Dinner | Snacks |
|--------|--------|
|        |        |

| Supplements | Medication |
|-------------|------------|
|             |            |

Date .................................................................................

Sleep quality and duration ....................................................

Stress levels    1   2   3   4   5   6   7   8   9   10

| Time | Systolic | Diastolic | Heart Rate |
|------|----------|-----------|------------|
|      |          |           |            |
|      |          |           |            |
|      |          |           |            |
|      |          |           |            |
|      |          |           |            |

Exercise and daily activities

Water Intake ▢▢▢▢▢▢▢

| Breakfast | Lunch |
|-----------|-------|
|           |       |

| Dinner | Snacks |
|--------|--------|
|        |        |

| Supplements | Medication |
|-------------|------------|
|             |            |

Date ....................................................................................................

Sleep quality and duration ............................................................

Stress levels     1    2    3    4    5    6    7    8    9    10

| Time | Systolic | Diastolic | Heart Rate |
|------|----------|-----------|------------|
|      |          |           |            |
|      |          |           |            |
|      |          |           |            |
|      |          |           |            |
|      |          |           |            |

Exercise and daily activities      Water Intake ☐☐☐☐☐☐☐

| Breakfast | Lunch |
|-----------|-------|
|           |       |

| Dinner | Snacks |
|--------|--------|
|        |        |

| Supplements | Medication |
|-------------|------------|
|             |            |

Date .............................................................................................

Sleep quality and duration ...................................................................

Stress levels     1   2   3   4   5   6   7   8   9   10

| Time | Systolic | Diastolic | Heart Rate |
|---|---|---|---|
|  |  |  |  |
|  |  |  |  |
|  |  |  |  |
|  |  |  |  |
|  |  |  |  |

Exercise and daily activities       Water Intake

| Breakfast | Lunch |
|---|---|
|  |  |
| Dinner | Snacks |
|  |  |
| Supplements | Medication |
|  |  |

Date .................................................................................................

Sleep quality and duration .........................................................

Stress levels      1    2    3    4    5    6    7    8    9    10

| Time | Systolic | Diastolic | Heart Rate |
|------|----------|-----------|------------|
|      |          |           |            |
|      |          |           |            |
|      |          |           |            |
|      |          |           |            |
|      |          |           |            |

Exercise and daily activities      Water Intake

| Breakfast | Lunch |
|-----------|-------|
|           |       |
| Dinner | Snacks |
|        |        |
| Supplements | Medication |
|             |            |

Date .................................................................................................

Sleep quality and duration .......................................................................

Stress levels     1    2    3    4    5    6    7    8    9    10

| Time | Systolic | Diastolic | Heart Rate |
|------|----------|-----------|------------|
|      |          |           |            |
|      |          |           |            |
|      |          |           |            |
|      |          |           |            |
|      |          |           |            |

Exercise and daily activities      Water Intake ☐☐☐☐☐☐☐

| Breakfast | Lunch |
|-----------|-------|
|           |       |

| Dinner | Snacks |
|--------|--------|
|        |        |

| Supplements | Medication |
|-------------|------------|
|             |            |

Date .............................................................................................................

Sleep quality and duration ...............................................................

Stress levels      1    2    3    4    5    6    7    8    9    10

| Time | Systolic | Diastolic | Heart Rate |
|------|----------|-----------|------------|
|      |          |           |            |
|      |          |           |            |
|      |          |           |            |
|      |          |           |            |
|      |          |           |            |

Exercise and daily activities      Water Intake

| Breakfast | Lunch |
|-----------|-------|
|           |       |

| Dinner | Snacks |
|--------|--------|
|        |        |

| Supplements | Medication |
|-------------|------------|
|             |            |

Date .................................................................................

Sleep quality and duration ...............................................

Stress levels      1    2    3    4    5    6    7    8    9    10

| Time | Systolic | Diastolic | Heart Rate |
|------|----------|-----------|------------|
|      |          |           |            |
|      |          |           |            |
|      |          |           |            |
|      |          |           |            |
|      |          |           |            |

Exercise and daily activities      Water Intake

| Breakfast | Lunch |
|-----------|-------|
|           |       |

| Dinner | Snacks |
|--------|--------|
|        |        |

| Supplements | Medication |
|-------------|------------|
|             |            |

Date .................................................................................................................

Sleep quality and duration .......................................................................

Stress levels          1     2     3     4     5     6     7     8     9     10

| Time | Systolic | Diastolic | Heart Rate |
|------|----------|-----------|------------|
|      |          |           |            |
|      |          |           |            |
|      |          |           |            |
|      |          |           |            |

Exercise and daily activities          Water Intake

| Breakfast | Lunch |
|-----------|-------|
|           |       |
| Dinner | Snacks |
|        |        |
| Supplements | Medication |
|             |            |

Date  ...........................................................................................................

Sleep quality and duration  .......................................................................

Stress levels     1    2    3    4    5    6    7    8    9    10

| Time | Systolic | Diastolic | Heart Rate |
|---|---|---|---|
|  |  |  |  |
|  |  |  |  |
|  |  |  |  |
|  |  |  |  |
|  |  |  |  |

Exercise and daily activities      Water Intake ⬜⬜⬜⬜⬜⬜⬜

| Breakfast | Lunch |
|---|---|
|  |  |
| Dinner | Snacks |
|  |  |
| Supplements | Medication |
|  |  |

Date ...........................................................................................

Sleep quality and duration ...................................................................

Stress levels     1    2    3    4    5    6    7    8    9    10

| Time | Systolic | Diastolic | Heart Rate |
|------|----------|-----------|------------|
|      |          |           |            |
|      |          |           |            |
|      |          |           |            |
|      |          |           |            |
|      |          |           |            |

Exercise and daily activities          Water Intake

...........................................................

...........................................................

...........................................................

...........................................................

...........................................................

...........................................................

...........................................................

...........................................................

...........................................................

...........................................................

...........................................................

...........................................................

...........................................................

| Breakfast | Lunch |
|-----------|-------|
|           |       |

| Dinner | Snacks |
|--------|--------|
|        |        |

| Supplements | Medication |
|-------------|------------|
|             |            |

Date ..........................................................................................................

Sleep quality and duration ......................................................................

Stress levels     1    2    3    4    5    6    7    8    9    10

| Time | Systolic | Diastolic | Heart Rate |
|---|---|---|---|
|  |  |  |  |
|  |  |  |  |
|  |  |  |  |
|  |  |  |  |
|  |  |  |  |

**Exercise and daily activities**      Water Intake

..........................................................
..........................................................
..........................................................
..........................................................
..........................................................
..........................................................
..........................................................
..........................................................
..........................................................
..........................................................
..........................................................
..........................................................
..........................................................
..........................................................
..........................................................
..........................................................

| Breakfast | Lunch |
|---|---|
|  |  |

| Dinner | Snacks |
|---|---|
|  |  |

| Supplements | Medication |
|---|---|
|  |  |

Date .........................................................................................................

Sleep quality and duration ............................................................................

Stress levels      1    2    3    4    5    6    7    8    9    10

| Time | Systolic | Diastolic | Heart Rate |
|---|---|---|---|
|  |  |  |  |
|  |  |  |  |
|  |  |  |  |
|  |  |  |  |
|  |  |  |  |

Exercise and daily activities      Water Intake

| Breakfast | Lunch |
|---|---|
|  |  |
| Dinner | Snacks |
|  |  |
| Supplements | Medication |
|  |  |

Date .........................................................................................................

Sleep quality and duration ....................................................................

Stress levels     1    2    3    4    5    6    7    8    9    10

| Time | Systolic | Diastolic | Heart Rate |
|------|----------|-----------|------------|
|      |          |           |            |
|      |          |           |            |
|      |          |           |            |
|      |          |           |            |
|      |          |           |            |

Exercise and daily activities     Water Intake ☐☐☐☐☐☐☐

| Breakfast | Lunch |
|-----------|-------|
|           |       |

| Dinner | Snacks |
|--------|--------|
|        |        |

| Supplements | Medication |
|-------------|------------|
|             |            |

Date .................................................................................................

Sleep quality and duration ...........................................................

Stress levels     1    2    3    4    5    6    7    8    9    10

| Time | Systolic | Diastolic | Heart Rate |
|---|---|---|---|
|  |  |  |  |
|  |  |  |  |
|  |  |  |  |
|  |  |  |  |
|  |  |  |  |

Exercise and daily activities      Water Intake

| Breakfast | Lunch |
|---|---|
|  |  |
| Dinner | Snacks |
|  |  |
| Supplements | Medication |
|  |  |

Date .........................................................................................................

Sleep quality and duration ...........................................................................

Stress levels      1    2    3    4    5    6    7    8    9    10

| Time | Systolic | Diastolic | Heart Rate |
|------|----------|-----------|------------|
|      |          |           |            |
|      |          |           |            |
|      |          |           |            |
|      |          |           |            |
|      |          |           |            |

Exercise and daily activities      Water Intake ☐☐☐☐☐☐☐☐

| Breakfast | Lunch |
|-----------|-------|
|           |       |

| Dinner | Snacks |
|--------|--------|
|        |        |

| Supplements | Medication |
|-------------|------------|
|             |            |

Date ...................................................................................................................................

Sleep quality and duration ...........................................................................................

Stress levels     1    2    3    4    5    6    7    8    9    10

| Time | Systolic | Diastolic | Heart Rate |
|---|---|---|---|
|  |  |  |  |
|  |  |  |  |
|  |  |  |  |
|  |  |  |  |
|  |  |  |  |

Exercise and daily activities      Water Intake

| Breakfast | Lunch |
|---|---|
|  |  |
| Dinner | Snacks |
|  |  |
| Supplements | Medication |
|  |  |

Date .................................................................................................

Sleep quality and duration ...................................................................

Stress levels     1   2   3   4   5   6   7   8   9   10

| Time | Systolic | Diastolic | Heart Rate |
|---|---|---|---|
|  |  |  |  |
|  |  |  |  |
|  |  |  |  |
|  |  |  |  |
|  |  |  |  |

Exercise and daily activities     Water Intake

..................................................

..................................................

..................................................

..................................................

..................................................

..................................................

..................................................

..................................................

..................................................

..................................................

..................................................

..................................................

..................................................

..................................................

..................................................

| Breakfast | Lunch |
|---|---|
|  |  |
| Dinner | Snacks |
|  |  |
| Supplements | Medication |
|  |  |

Date  ...........................................................................................................

Sleep quality and duration  ...........................................................................

Stress levels      1    2    3    4    5    6    7    8    9    10

| Time | Systolic | Diastolic | Heart Rate |
|------|----------|-----------|------------|
|      |          |           |            |
|      |          |           |            |
|      |          |           |            |
|      |          |           |            |
|      |          |           |            |

**Exercise and daily activities**　　　　Water Intake ☐☐☐☐☐☐☐

| Breakfast | Lunch |
|-----------|-------|
|           |       |

| Dinner | Snacks |
|--------|--------|
|        |        |

| Supplements | Medication |
|-------------|------------|
|             |            |

Date .......................................................................................................................

Sleep quality and duration ..............................................................................

Stress levels      1    2    3    4    5    6    7    8    9    10

| Time | Systolic | Diastolic | Heart Rate |
|------|----------|-----------|------------|
|      |          |           |            |
|      |          |           |            |
|      |          |           |            |
|      |          |           |            |
|      |          |           |            |

Exercise and daily activities        Water Intake

........................................................

........................................................

........................................................

........................................................

........................................................

........................................................

........................................................

........................................................

........................................................

........................................................

........................................................

........................................................

........................................................

........................................................

........................................................

| Breakfast | Lunch |
|-----------|-------|
|           |       |

| Dinner | Snacks |
|--------|--------|
|        |        |

| Supplements | Medication |
|-------------|------------|
|             |            |

Date .........................................................................................................

Sleep quality and duration .............................................................

Stress levels     1    2    3    4    5    6    7    8    9    10

| Time | Systolic | Diastolic | Heart Rate |
|------|----------|-----------|------------|
|      |          |           |            |
|      |          |           |            |
|      |          |           |            |
|      |          |           |            |
|      |          |           |            |

Exercise and daily activities      Water Intake

| Breakfast | Lunch |
|-----------|-------|
|           |       |

| Dinner | Snacks |
|--------|--------|
|        |        |

| Supplements | Medication |
|-------------|------------|
|             |            |

Date .............................................................................................................

Sleep quality and duration ...............................................................

Stress levels     1   2   3   4   5   6   7   8   9   10

| Time | Systolic | Diastolic | Heart Rate |
|------|----------|-----------|------------|
|      |          |           |            |
|      |          |           |            |
|      |          |           |            |
|      |          |           |            |
|      |          |           |            |

Exercise and daily activities    Water Intake

| Breakfast | Lunch |
|-----------|-------|
|           |       |

| Dinner | Snacks |
|--------|--------|
|        |        |

| Supplements | Medication |
|-------------|------------|
|             |            |

Date ...................................................................................................................

Sleep quality and duration ...................................................................................

Stress levels      1    2    3    4    5    6    7    8    9    10

| Time | Systolic | Diastolic | Heart Rate |
|---|---|---|---|
|  |  |  |  |
|  |  |  |  |
|  |  |  |  |
|  |  |  |  |
|  |  |  |  |

Exercise and daily activities      Water Intake

| Breakfast | Lunch |
|---|---|
|  |  |
| Dinner | Snacks |
|  |  |
| Supplements | Medication |
|  |  |

Date .........................................................................................................

Sleep quality and duration ...............................................................

Stress levels      1    2    3    4    5    6    7    8    9    10

| Time | Systolic | Diastolic | Heart Rate |
|---|---|---|---|
|  |  |  |  |
|  |  |  |  |
|  |  |  |  |
|  |  |  |  |
|  |  |  |  |

**Exercise and daily activities**      **Water Intake**

| Breakfast | Lunch |
|---|---|
|  |  |
| Dinner | Snacks |
|  |  |
| Supplements | Medication |
|  |  |

Date ..........................................................................................................

Sleep quality and duration ........................................................................

Stress levels     1   2   3   4   5   6   7   8   9   10

| Time | Systolic | Diastolic | Heart Rate |
|------|----------|-----------|------------|
|      |          |           |            |
|      |          |           |            |
|      |          |           |            |
|      |          |           |            |
|      |          |           |            |

Exercise and daily activities      Water Intake

| Breakfast | Lunch |
|-----------|-------|
|           |       |

| Dinner | Snacks |
|--------|--------|
|        |        |

| Supplements | Medication |
|-------------|------------|
|             |            |

Date .................................................................................................

Sleep quality and duration ................................................................

Stress levels    1   2   3   4   5   6   7   8   9   10

| Time | Systolic | Diastolic | Heart Rate |
|---|---|---|---|
|  |  |  |  |
|  |  |  |  |
|  |  |  |  |
|  |  |  |  |
|  |  |  |  |

Exercise and daily activities     Water Intake

| Breakfast | Lunch |
|---|---|
|  |  |
| Dinner | Snacks |
|  |  |
| Supplements | Medication |
|  |  |

Date .........................................................................................................

Sleep quality and duration .........................................................................

Stress levels     1    2    3    4    5    6    7    8    9    10

| Time | Systolic | Diastolic | Heart Rate |
|------|----------|-----------|------------|
|      |          |           |            |
|      |          |           |            |
|      |          |           |            |
|      |          |           |            |
|      |          |           |            |

Exercise and daily activities      Water Intake

| Breakfast | Lunch |
|-----------|-------|
|           |       |

| Dinner | Snacks |
|--------|--------|
|        |        |

| Supplements | Medication |
|-------------|------------|
|             |            |

www.ingramcontent.com/pod-product-compliance
Lightning Source LLC
Chambersburg PA
CBHW040144110726
48005CB00018B/2640